IN SICKNESS AND IN HEALTH

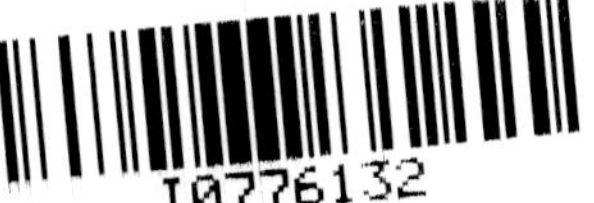

Donald Gorbach

ISBN:1977605435
ISBN-13: 978-1977605436

"IT'S NOT HOW YOU FEEL, IT'S HOW YOU LOOK
AND YOU LOOK MAHVELOUS"

-BILLY CRYSTAL

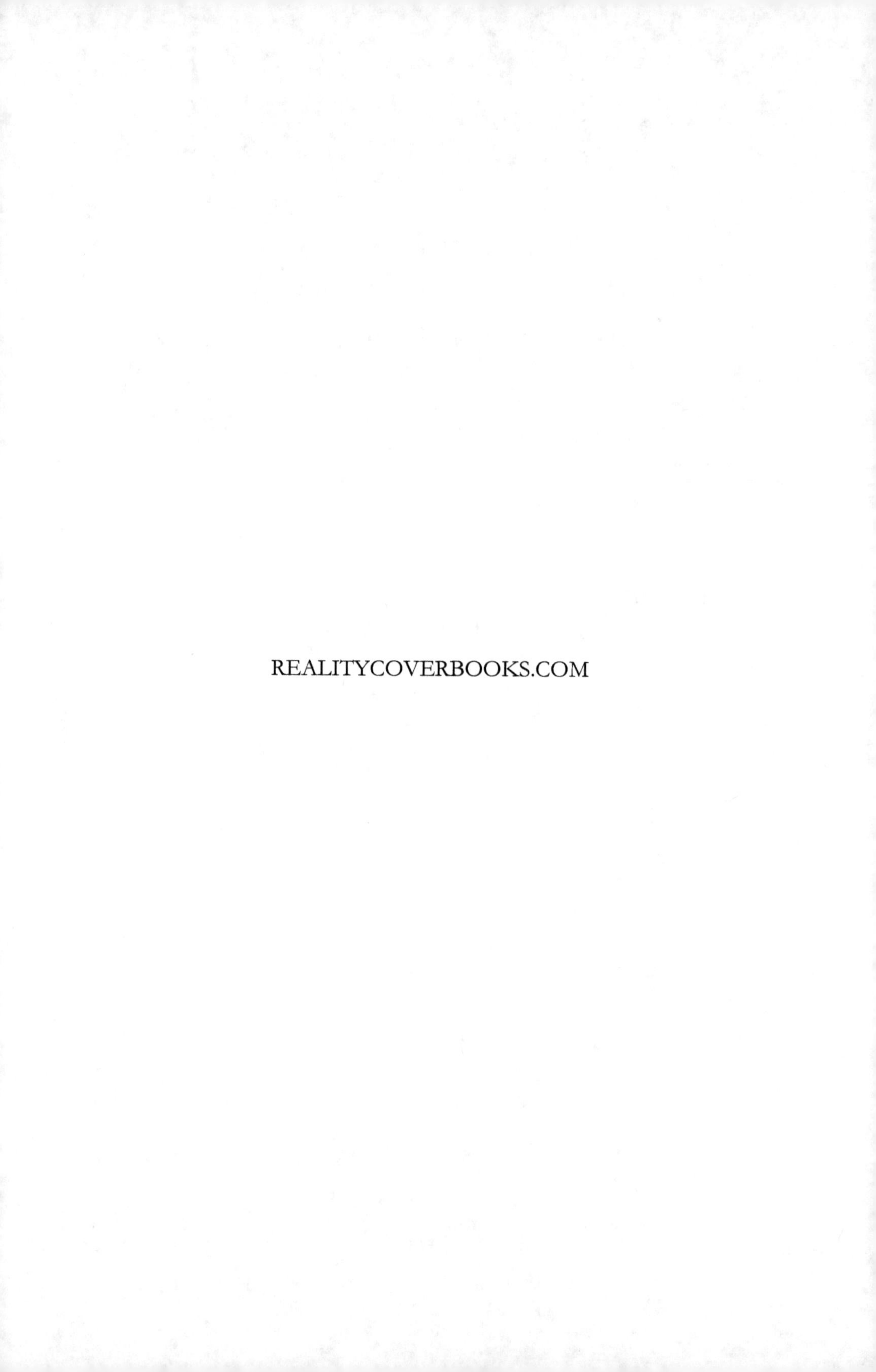

REALITYCOVERBOOKS.COM